Mariem TURKI
Imen CHAARI
Jihen ALOULOU

PRESCRIBING HYPNOTICS TO ELDERLY PATIENTS IN GENERAL MEDICINE

Mariem TURKI
Imen CHAARI
Jihen ALOULOU

PRESCRIBING HYPNOTICS TO ELDERLY PATIENTS IN GENERAL MEDICINE

ScienciaScripts

Imprint

Cover image: www.ingimage.com

This book is a translation from the original published under ISBN 978-620-6-72034-8.

Publisher:
Sciencia Scripts
is a trademark of
Dodo Books Indian Ocean Ltd. and OmniScriptum S.R.L publishing group

120 High Road, East Finchley, London, N2 9ED, United Kingdom
Str. Armeneasca 28/1, office 1, Chisinau MD-2012, Republic of Moldova, Europe
Printed at: see last page
ISBN: 978-620-8-04123-6

PRESCRIBING HYPNOTICS TO ELDERLY PATIENTS IN GENERAL MEDICINE

SUMMARY INTRODUCTION

Insomnia is one of the most common reasons for prescribing psychotropic drugs to the elderly. Management of insomnia must take account of age-related physiological changes, more frequent co-morbidities and multiple medications.

OBJECTIVE

To evaluate GP practices in the management of insomnia in AS and compare them with international recommendations.

POPULATION AND METHODS

This was an observational, cross-sectional, descriptive study of 32 general practitioners in the Sfax region (Tunisia), using an online questionnaire.

RESULTS

Among the participants, 62.5% reported that they are very often or often called upon by patients consulting them for insomnia. Before prescribing a hypnotic, 65.6% of doctors reported that they usually advise patients to follow certain dietary hygiene rules. The most commonly used classes of hypnotics were: benzodiazepines (BZDs) 59.37%; antihistamines 59.37%; homeopathic treatments 56.25% and phytotherapy 50%. The examples of prescriptions proposed by the participants showed that the duration of treatment was not in line with international recommendations in 18.75% of cases. As for the prescription of BZDs, half-life molecules were used in 37.48% of cases, the dosage was identical to that for adults in 34.4% of cases, and the withdrawal syndrome was unknown in 56.25% of cases.

CONCLUSION

Prescribing a hypnotic treatment for the elderly is a logical approach to care, following a precise diagnosis and taking into account psychiatric and somatic comorbidities, precautions for use and contraindications. In this context, we have highlighted a number of shortcomings in the management of insomnia in elderly patients in general practice. There is a need for more training in this area.

1. INTRODUCTION

Sleep disorders are one of the most common reasons for prescribing psychotropic drugs to elderly patients. Insomnia, defined as difficulties falling asleep or staying asleep, or non-restorative sleep, is the most common sleep disorder in this age group, with a prevalence ranging from 30% to 48% [1].

Indeed, advancing age modifies sleep physiology. As a result, some insomnia is not necessarily pathological, and is instead explained by physiological ageing. However, several pathological processes, both somatic and psychiatric, as well as environmental disturbances, may coexist, resulting in what is known as secondary insomnia.

The management of sleep complaints in the elderly must take into account the physiological changes associated with age, the greater frequency of co-morbidities and the multiple medications used. Hypnotics must therefore be prescribed with caution, as they are particularly likely to cause falls in the elderly, with sometimes serious complications, as well as cognitive impairment and road accidents. In order to minimise these risks, prescriptions must comply with international recommendations.

The prescription of psychotropic drugs (anxiolytics, hypnotics, neuroleptics, antidepressants, etc.) is a major and complex health problem, particularly in the AS population. Numerous studies [2-4] have highlighted the high incidence of psychotropic drug misuse and the need for targeted action, particularly in the highly exposed and vulnerable AS population. Moreover, in 2008, the French National Authority for Health (HAS), in its"Between September and December 2007 in France, 32% of people aged over 65 and almost 40% of people aged over 85 were prescribed a hypnotic or anxiolytic" [5].

It follows that optimising prescriptions for ADTs is a major public health issue. In this context, the GP is in the best position to investigate and manage AS sleep complaints. Referral to specialists may then be essential, either to advance the diagnosis and management of associated somatic and/or psychiatric illnesses, or to explore a sleep pathology. The aim of this study was to assess how general practitioners manage insomnia in AS and to analyse whether there is a gap between this management and international recommendations.

2. POPULATION AND METHODS

2.1. Type of study :

We conducted an observational, cross-sectional, descriptive study of professional practice in the management of patients with ADHD who suffer from insomnia among general practitioners.

2.2. Sample

2.2.1. Inclusion criteria :

General practitioners in the Sfax region (Tunisia), practising in the public and private sectors, who agreed to take part in the study.

2.2.2. Exclusion criteria :

Doctors working in emergency units.

2.3. study protocol

We invited doctors to take part in our survey by sending them a questionnaire by e-mail, which they completed anonymously.

The questionnaire was produced using a web-based programme called "Google Forms", which enables it to be presented in a clear, easy-to-complete format. Responses are collected automatically and anonymously.

The questionnaire is preceded by a message explaining the framework of the study and thanking the doctor for his cooperation.

This questionnaire includes :

- 6 items specifying sociodemographic characteristics and data on the doctor's professional activity.
- 13 items specifying the place of sleep complaints among consultations by the

elderly: frequency; explorations; hygienic and dietary rules; psychotropic drugs used.

- 6 items exploring the last prescription issued to an elderly person for the treatment of insomnia. These items assess the hypnotic used (molecule, dosage, duration) and the other treatments prescribed (in order to explore the presence of any drug interactions).
- 6 items relating to the prescription of benzodiazepines: molecules; dosage; contraindications; side effects; withdrawal.
- Finally, there are 2 last items in which the doctor expresses a possible request for training in this area.

A total of 348 e-mails were sent. In addition to the first mailing, two further reminders were sent at 15-day intervals.

2.4. Analysis statistics

Statistical analysis was carried out using the Windows Statistical Package for Social Sciences (SPSS 20). Quantitative variables were expressed as means and standard deviations, while qualitative variables were expressed in terms of numbers and proportions.

3. RESULTS

3.1.Rate of responses

Out of a total of 348 e-mails sent, we only received 32 responses, a response rate of 9.2%.

3.2.Results descriptive

3.2.1. Profile of prescribing doctors

The majority of doctors who responded to the questionnaire were men: 56.2% versus 43.75%, giving an M/F sex ratio of 1.28 (Figure 1). The mean age was 45.21 ± 10.71 years (min: 28; max: 64). The age range was between 35 and 49 years in 43.75% of cases (Figure 2).

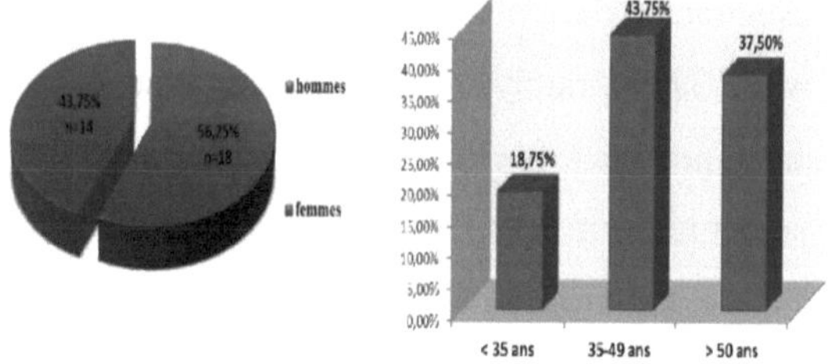

Figure 1: breakdown of participants by gender

Figure 2: age distribution of participants

The average number of years worked was 15.4 ± 10.12 years (min: 1; max: 34 years).46.9% of patients worked in rural areas and 53.1% in urban areas. More than half of the doctors (56.3%) worked in the public sector. In the course of their training, 40.6% of doctors reported having received training in geriatrics, the breakdown of which is as follows (table T):

Table I: Training received in health care for the elderly

Type of training	n	%
A master's degree or postgraduate diploma in geriatrics	8	25
CEC (Certificate of Complementary Studies) psychogeriatrics	1	3,12
Pharmacogeriatric CEC	1	3,12
Continuing medical education	3	9,38
No training	19	59,38

3.2.2. Insomnia in elderly patients in general practice

Of the participants, 12.5% reported that they are very often approached by SAs consulting for insomnia, 50% reported that they often receive elderly patients with insomnia, while 37.5% rarely meet them.The doctors reported an average of 3.43 consultations per week for this reason (min 1, max 15). This complaint came from the patient himself in 46.87% of cases, from the spouse or family in 46.87% of cases, and was noted in the course of the medical history in 6.25% of cases.

The half of doctors had reported not request any additional tests when faced with an isolated sleep complaint. However, the others had indicated systematic explorations, distributed as follows (table TT):

Table II: Complementary tests ordered for insomnia in older people

Explorations		n	%
Biological tests	CBC (blood count)	7	21,87
	Inflammatory assessment	5	15,62
	Renal check-up	8	25
	Blood glucose	6	18,75
	Lipid balance	5	15,62
	ECBU (Cytobacteriological Examination of the urine)	2	6,25
	Hormone check-up	6	18,75
	total	13	40,62
Radiological investigations	Brain scan	2	6,25
	Chest X-ray	1	3,12
	total	3	9,37
ECG (Electro-Cardio-Gram)		1	3,12
Neuro-psychological investigations (mini GDS; MMSE (Mini Mental State Examination))		1	3,12

3.2.3. Medical prescriptions

- **Hygienic and dietetic rules**

Among our participants, 65.6% reported having the habit of advising a few dietary hygiene rules before prescribing a hypnotic. These rules are detailed in the table TTT :

Table III: The main health and diet rules proposed by participants

Rules	n	%
Avoid stimulants in the evening	16	50
Avoid sleeping during the day, reduce the length of naps	8	25
Do some physical activity during the day	5	15,62
Respect sleep schedules	6	18,75
Avoid heavy meals at night	5	15,62
Avoid eating late	4	12,5
Ensuring a comfortable night's sleep	5	15,62
Do not change your bed or pillow	1	3,12
Not sleeping very early	1	3,12
Take an herbal tea before bed	1	3,12
Read a book before going to sleep	1	3,12

For 28.1% of participants, these rules would often be effective. However, 53.1% thought they would rarely be effective and 18.8% thought they would never be effective.

Prescribing hypnotics

Over a third (34.4%) of doctors reported that they found it easy to prescribe a hypnotic for an elderly patient. In 12.5% of cases, this prescription was made during the first consultation. The most commonly used therapeutic classes were as follows (Figure 3)

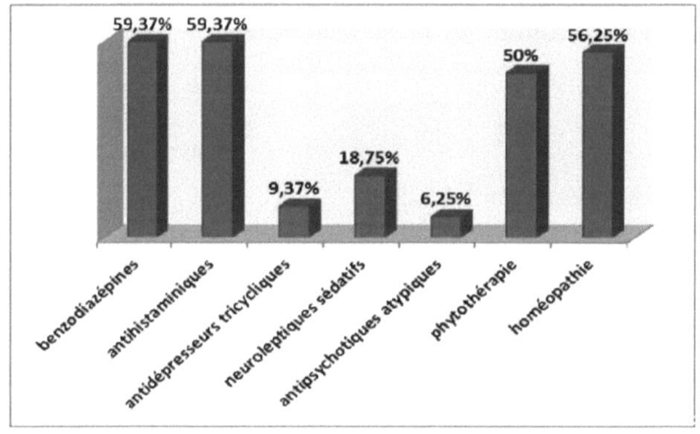

Figure 3: Classes of sleeping pills used by GPs

In addition, 40.6% thought they had control over the prescribing of hypnotics for AS, which would be done in accordance with the recommendations in ¼ of cases. However, 46.9% said they were unaware of these recommendations. Non-compliance with these recommendations was explained by the time constraints involved in consulting them in 31.3% of cases. Thus, 46.9% of doctors often referred patients to a psychiatrist.

3.2.3. Details of last prescription

- **Patient data :**

More than half of all hypnotic prescriptions were for women (62.5%), with an average age of 71.9. The average age for men was 75. For both sexes, the average age was 73.15.± 8.17 years.

- **The context of the prescription** :

In most cases (71.9%), this was a first prescription. The indication was occasional insomnia in half the cases, chronic insomnia in 31.25% of cases and insomnia related to a mental or physical pathology in 18.75% of cases. Figures 4 and 5 summarise the different classes of drugs prescribed. Benzodiazepines

(BZDs) were the most commonly prescribed drugs.

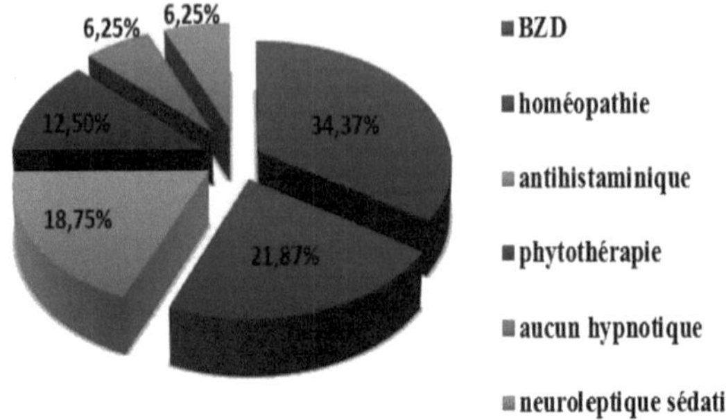

Figure 4: Classes of drugs prescribed when last prescribed

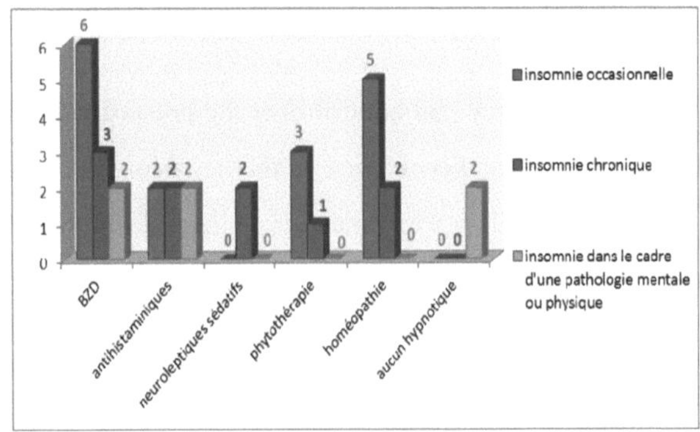

Figure 5: Distribution of hypnotics prescribed according to the context of insomnia

Prescription period

The average duration of prescription was 29.53 ± 20.66 days, with extremes ranging from 7 to 90 days. A treatment duration exceeding 30 days was noted in 18.75% of prescriptions. Figure 6 shows the duration of hypnotic treatment according to the type of insomnia.

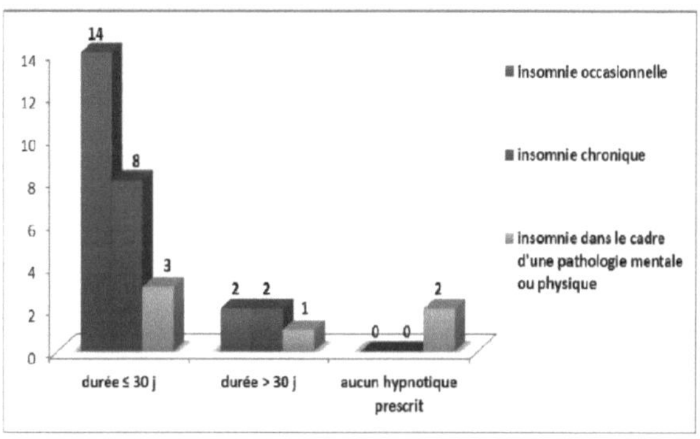

Figure 6: Breakdown of the duration of treatment according to the treatment context insomnia

Associated treatments :

The following figure (Figure 7) shows the profile of the different prescriptions proposed.

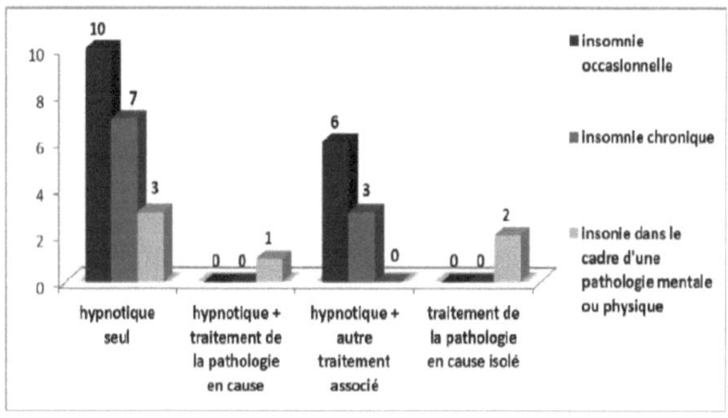

Figure 7: **distribution of drug prescriptions according to the context of insomnia**

Moreover, among these prescriptions, we noted a combination of 2 hypnotics in 6.37% of cases.

3.2.4. Prescribing benzodiazepines and related substances

The molecules used

Figure 8 shows the most commonly used molecules:

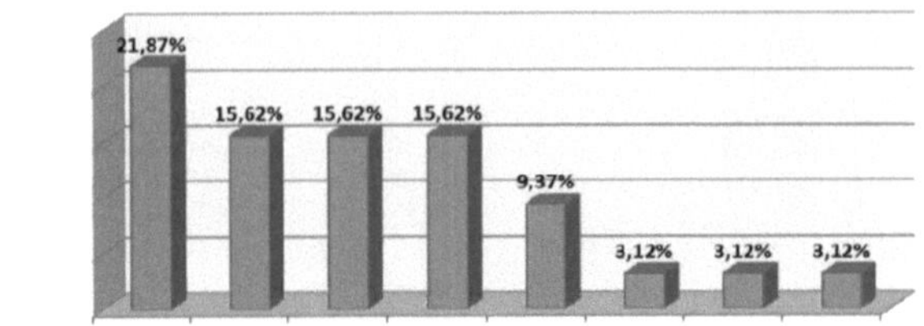

figure 8: the different BZDs and related products used

Half-life :

Long half-life BZDs (lexomil®; lysanxia®; tranxene®; valium®) were used in 37.48% of cases.Eighteen point eight per cent of doctors reported using molecules with a long half-life and 40.6% with a short half-life. However, ¼ of them did not know the half-life of the compounds they used.

Dosage:

The dosage was half that for adults in 28.1% of cases, and identical in 34.4% of cases. However, 37.5% did not know the recommended dosage.

Drug combinations :

Of the prescriptions proposed that included a BZD (n=11), a combination of drugs was noted in 45.45% of cases (n=5). The various treatments associated with BZDs were: insulin; iron; calcium; risperidone; aspirin; captopril; non-steroidal anti-inflammatory drugs; and a second BZD.

Contraindications:

Before prescribing BZDs, 75% of participants recognised the contraindications to be eliminated. The most frequently reported are shown in Table TV:

Table IV: Contraindications to the use of BZDs reported by participants

Contraindications	n	%
Severe respiratory insufficiency	19	59,3
Sleep apnoea syndrome	6	18,75
Liver failure	9	28,12
myasthenia	5	15,62
allergy	3	9,37
Renal insufficiency	5	15,62
Heart failure	3	9,37
pregnancy	1	3,12
Don't know	8	25

- **Side effects:**

The side effects reported by 59.37% of doctors were (Table V):

Table V: Main side-effects associated with the use of BZDs reported by participants

Undesirable effects	n	%
Drowsiness/sedation	7	21,87
Behavioural problems/agitation	3	9,37
Asthenia	2	6,25
Risk of falling	1	3,12
Risk of road accidents	1	3,12
Memory disorders	2	6,25
Respiratory problems	2	6,25
dependency	3	9,37
headaches	1	3,12
vomiting	1	3,12
Don't know	13	40,6

In cases of intractable insomnia, 43.8% of doctors combined a BZD with another hypnotic and 25% referred the patient to a psychiatrist.

- **Weaning :**

  - The average duration after which weaning was envisaged was 50 days of treatment (from 15 days to 6 months). This duration exceeded 30 days in half of the cases.
  - The ability of elderly patients to stop taking BZDs was not recognised by any of the doctors.
  - The average duration of withdrawal was 47 days, with extremes ranging from

7 days to 6 months. In 18.75% of cases, weaning was completed in less than 30 days.

o During and/or after withdrawal, 12.5% of doctors systematically substituted the BZD with another hypnotic of a different class.

o The most frequently reported signs of withdrawal syndrome were (Figure 9):

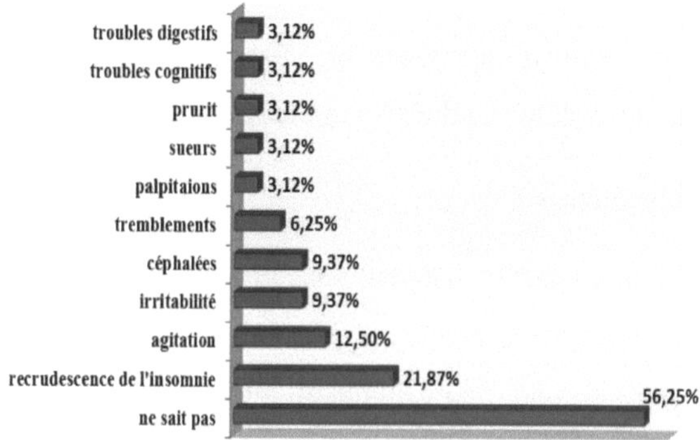

Figure 9: Symptoms of withdrawal syndrome reported by doctors

o To curb this syndrome, the participants proposed the following actions:

• Substitution by a non-BZD hypnotic: 9.37

• Symptomatic treatment with beta-blockers: 3.12

• Return to previous dose: 3.12

• Look for anxiety/depression: 3.12%.

• Referral to psychiatrist 6.25

However, 62.5% of doctors did not report any conduct.

3.2.5. General impressions

At after the questionnaire, 78,1% had looking forwardà read the recommendations for the management of insomnia in AS.The majority of participants (93.8%) said they needed training on this subject.

4. DISCUSSION

4.1. Insomnia in the elderly

4.1.1. Sleep patterns in the elderly

4.1.1.1. Factors modifying the sleep-wake rhythm

The nycthemeral rhythm is influenced by internal and external synchronisers, both of which are altered during the ageing process:

- **Internal synchronizers** :

Tls include hormonal factors (melatonin, growth hormone (GH), cortisol, adrenalin and noradrenalin), as well as internal temperature [6]. With ageing, several morphological and neurochemical alterations occur in the centres responsible for endogenous circadian regulation. Melatonin is a natural hormone produced by the pineal gland (epiphysis) which is an endogenous sleep inducer. Melatonin synthesis in the elderly is reduced in only a few people [7], but its secretion decreases more rapidly over the course of the day than in young people [6].

✓ GH is synthesised during deep slow wave sleep (FLS). Its level of production becomes very low in the elderly and parallels the decrease in LPS [6]. Cortisol secretion levels increase with age. Its peak secretions are thought to correlate with the onset of nocturnal wakefulness [8].

✓ Adrenalin and noradrenalin levels increase with age, but retain their circadian rhythm. Their increase is also correlated with increased nocturnal wakefulness.

✓ Internal temperature, another synchroniser, is about an hour ahead of phase. In addition, the amplitude of the temperature rhythm in elderly subjects is 20 to 30% lower than in younger subjects. Finally, the propensity to wake up closer to the thermal minimum increases with age [9,10].

✦ **External synchronizers** :

These include the light-dark cycle, physical activity, hours of rest and so-called social factors, which include mealtimes, waking times and bedtimes [6,11].

In AS, the influence of these synchronisers is reduced. In fact, there is a reduction in daytime physical activity, little exposure to temperature variations, mealtimes and bedtimes that are too early, and little exposure to light [6].

4.1.1.2. Sleep organisation in the elderly

Physiological ageing can be accompanied by certain architectural changes in sleep. The ability to remain asleep is altered by ageing, the number of awakenings and their duration increases with age, but the ability to fall asleep is not modified. Only the ability to go back to sleep is altered. The reappearance of naps, and often their excessive duration, aggravates the poor quality of night-time sleep, reducing its length. These factors contribute to the circadian changes observed in the elderly, in whom the agendas of the day and night are not always the same. Sleep and actimetric readings show the gradual development of polyphasic, phase-advanced sleep [6]. Studies of polysomnographic tracings have revealed several hypnographic structural elements [12].

✦ sleep efficiency lowered to 80-85% of Total Sleep Time [9]. decrease in Deep Slow Sleep [13-15], mainly in men.concomitant increase in Light Slow Sleep [15];

- little quantitative variation in Paradoxical Sleep (PS) but with a shorter onset latency. The phases of PS are more fragmented, their duration is reduced [16], and they tend to be equal throughout the night [13];
- an increase in the number and duration of awakenings during sleep, more frequently in the second half of the night;
- very significant increase in sleep microfractionation ;
- sleep instability, with more frequent changes in sleep stage.

These factors shed light on the perception of choppy, less recuperative sleep described by older people.

4.1.2. Definition of insomnia

Insomnia is a subjective experience defined by difficulties in falling asleep or staying asleep, or non-restorative sleep. It is associated with daytime symptoms such as fatigue or drowsiness, problems with concentration and memory, gloominess or irritability, and sometimes a loss of motivation [17]. In fact, there are three international classifications which precisely define the various sleep disorders, in particular insomnia: the DSM-, the DSM-IV and the DSM-IV.5 (Diagnostic and Statistical Manual of Mental Disorders), the International Classification of Diseases (TCI-10) and the Classification of Mental Disorders (CMD-10). Tnternationale des Troubles du Sommeil (CTTS) (or TCSD (Tnternational Classification Of Sleep Disorders). For example, according to the DSM 5, 2 other criteria are required for the definition of "insomnia disorder": difficulty sleeping for at least 3 nights a week, and for at least 3 months.

4.1.3. Classification

According to the latest TCSD 3 edition in 2014, insomnia is classified into 3 main categories:

- **Chronic insomnia**

- Psychophysiologicalnsomnia - Paradoxicalnsomnia
- Idiopathic insomnia
- Tnsomnia due to mental illness
- Insomnia due to inadequate sleep hygiene - Behavioural insomnia in children
- Tnsomnia due to medication - Tnsomnia due to illness

- **Short-term insomnia**

- Tnsomnia of adjustment

- **Other types of insomnia**

4.1.4. Epidemiological data

Nearly half of people over 65 complain of sleep problems [18]. Although these complaints are common, they do not necessarily correspond to insomnia and do not always justify the use of a sleeping pill. Older people are more likely to be regular users of sleeping pills than younger people [19], yet hypnotics are rarely considered as medicines by the SA [20].The 2007 HAS publication on benzodiazepines in the elderly shows that the annual prevalence of hypnotic use varies from 12% to 15% for men and from 19% to 22% for women. In France, a quarter of people aged between 65 and 74 and a third of people over 74 take medication to help them sleep [21]. Our study showed that insomnia is a frequent complaint in the elderly. In fact, 62.5% of doctors reported that they were often or very often called upon by patients consulting them for insomnia.

2. Evaluation of the management of insomnia in AS by GPs (comparison with international recommendations)

In our study, more than half the doctors (59.4%) thought they had shortcomings in the management of insomnia, which seems to be linked to a lack of knowledge of the recommendations. GPs are generally poorly trained in this area. Indeed, nearly a third of them explained this by the time constraints involved in reading them. However, it is important to note that the majority were interested in reading the recommendations, which suggests that they are relevant and that the subject is important. Through the presentation of a summary of the HAS recommendations, which appeared in its reports "Improving the prescribing of psychotropic drugs in the elderly" [22] and "Stopping the use of benzodiazepines and related drugs in the elderly" [23] in October 2007; "Management of insomnia in general practice. Professional recommendations. 2007" [24] and "Arrêt des benzodiazépines et médicaments apparentés : démarche du médecin traitant en ambulatoire, Juin 2015" [25] we are going to highlight the gap in doctors' practices. When dealing with an AS presenting a complaint about sleep, the first thing to do is to make sure that the complaint is indeed insomnia. In addition to the sensation of sleeping badly, insomnia includes daytime repercussions such as fatigue, difficulty concentrating and impaired social functioning .

4.2.1. Sleep hygiene

Once the diagnosis has been made, the quality of sleep hygiene is an essential parameter to be specified. Among the participants in our study, 65.6% reported having the habit of advising a few hygienic and dietary rules before prescribing a hypnotic. This is in line with HAS recommendations. The latter insists that, in all cases, before any other initiative is taken, it is advisable to ensure that a few basic rules of sleep hygiene are met. These rules have been the subject of interest in several articles in the literature [3,11,26]. These rules consist of :

- Healthy eating and habits
- Limit stimulants (coffee, tea, fizzy drinks), especially 4 to 6 hours before bedtime
- Limiting alcohol and tobacco
- A light snack at bedtime can help induce sleep.
- Avoid large, fatty meals in the evening Eat at regular times;
- Prepare for sleep with 20 to 30 minutes of relaxation (soft music).
- Take a lukewarm bath to help lower the temperature needed to fall asleep
- Avoid activities stimulating just before the bedtime (television, computer, etc.)
- Adopt a regular waking schedule, avoid sleeping during the day after a bad night's sleep
- Sleep as required, but no more; avoid naps that are too long (> 1 hour) or too late (after 4pm).

- Maintaining regular activities

- Avoid physical activity for 4 to 6 hours before bedtime
- Moderate physical activity during the day helps to limit anxiety or mood disorders and helps you to fall asleep.
- Exposure to light

- Going out during the day if possible.

- Natural light in the morning by opening the bedroom shutters, especially if the person is bedridden;
- A room that meets certain requirements:

- Have a comfortable, cool bed, a well-ventilated, noise-free room, opaque curtains, etc.
- For bed-ridden people who often have the television in the room, find a solution to watch it in a position other than lying down.

According to the HAS, these rules can sometimes be sufficient to restore sleep in cases of mild insomnia without comorbidities. However, they are not sufficient on their own to solve the problem of insomnia. moderate or severe, in which case they should be combined with other therapeutic measures [27].

Moreover, 71.9% of participants reported that these rules are rarely or never effective on their own. Thus, if there is no improvement despite good sleep hygiene, the management of insomnia will depend on its context (appendix 1):

- If the insomnia is more occasional, sometimes with an identifiable stress factor, we are in the context of adjustment insomnia. In our study, this situation accounted for half of the prescriptions offered (n=16). In 50% of these prescriptions (n=8), phytotherapy or homeopathy was proposed. BZDs were prescribed for 37.5% of patients (n=6), and an antihistamine in 12.5% of cases (n=2). This is in line with HAS recommendations, which recommend that, if necessary, the most conservative symptomatic treatment possible should be offered: either a mild sedative (phytotherapy) or a hypnotic (doxylamine, BZD or related).

Whichever hypnotic is chosen, the lowest effective dose should be sought and prescribed for a limited period, from a few days to a maximum of 4 weeks. The duration of treatment (<30 days) was respected in 87.5% (n=14) of prescriptions for occasional insomnia in our study.

o Looking for signs associated with insomnia (chronic pain, depression, etc.) may point to a somatic and/or psychiatric co-morbidity. In our study, of the prescriptions proposed in this context (6 prescriptions, i.e. 18.75%), only 3 (9.37%) included treatment of the associated pathology, and in 2 of these, the treatment of this pathology was isolated (no associated sleeping pill). In the 4 cases where a hypnotic was indicated, it was prescribed on an occasional basis (<1 month) in 3 cases and for a prolonged period (>1 month) in the other case. According to According to the HAS, the treatment to be established for chronic insomnia with comorbidities depends on the associated pathology likely to cause, maintain or aggravate the insomnia. As a general rule, insomnia should be assessed and treated on its own merits, as treatment of associated disorders does not automatically lead to a return to sleep. The occasional prescription of low-dose hypnotics may prove useful, despite the lack of studies demonstrating their value.

4.2.2. Cognitive-behavioural therapies

In cases where insomnia is chronic and not associated with co-morbidities (31.25% of prescriptions), the participating doctors proposed a sleeping pill in all cases, with the duration of treatment being >30 days in only 20% of cases. The HAS stresses that the efficacy of prolonged treatment has not been demonstrated, as addiction may occur. Congenitive and Compensatory Therapies (CCT) are most appropriate here. They are the first-line treatment for chronic insomnia. Their efficacy has been well demonstrated in young subjects and those with AD [28,29]. They act on the factors that maintain insomnia by focusing on the psychological and behavioural components of insomnia. Their principles can easily be applied by general practitioners, in collaboration with psychiatrists and psychologists.

- **Sleep restriction** [11,30]

It consists of limiting the number of hours spent in bed quite strictly and according to very regular schedules. In this way, we are going to voluntarily induce relative sleep deprivation. This will have the effect of rapidly increasing the quality of sleep, reversing a situation where the patient was struggling to sleep (which is replaced by a situation in which he or she is struggling to stay awake) and to synchronise and reinforce the biological clock signal.

- **Stimulus control** [11]

Patients suffering from chronic insomnia often adopt behaviours that perpetuate the problems (watching television in bed, worrying about falling asleep). Stimulus control aims to eliminate these behaviours and reinforce the association between bedtime and sleep.

o Patients determine their bedtimes and wake-up times according to their physiological needs.

o The nap should last less than an hour and take place before 3pm o A pre-bedtime ritual for falling asleep should be established with the patient (e.g. relaxation for half an hour before bedtime or a warm bath 90 minutes before bedtime). o The bedroom should be comfortable and quiet, and reserved solely for sleeping. Conversely, patients should only sleep in their own bedrooms.

o If it is difficult to fall asleep, the subject will get up and go back to bed only when he or she feels the need to sleep.

- **Relaxation methods** [11]

The aim of relaxation is to guide the subject towards a state of tranquillity when he or she wishes to sleep. There are many different techniques:

- The most classic is Schulz's autogenic training, the aim of which is to establish automatisms that allow the subject to relax physically and mentally whatever the circumstances [31].

- progressive muscle relaxation (tension and release of each muscle) mental imagery training

- diaphragmatic breathing

- biofeedback.

- Yoga

- **Cognitive therapy** [11]

Aims to get patients to identify their astonishing beliefs, to consider alternative hypotheses and to change attitudes that are detrimental to sleep. It mainly involves :

- Avoid seeing insomnia as the cause of all the day's problems
- Don't overreact after a bad night's sleep; learn to tolerate insomnia
- Do not try to induce sleep on command
- Revising misconceptions about the causes of insomnia

- **Paradoxical intention** [11]

This consists of encouraging the patient to fight against sleep for as long as possible once in bed. The therapy seems difficult to implement because it is not well accepted by patients.

4.2.3. Prescription drugs

In our study, benzodiazepines were used in 59.37% of cases; phytotherapy 50%; homeopathy 56.25%; antihistamines 59.37%; sedative neuroleptics in 18.75% of cases and tricyclic antidepressants in 9.37% of cases. However, not all of these classes are appropriate for AS. In fact, greater caution is required, due to the fragility of the condition (altered pharmacokinetics, increased sensitivity of the central nervous system, drug interactions). The usual adverse effects of BZDs are more frequent, in particular the risk of falls or driving accidents and their attendant complications. Information on these The patient should be informed of the physiological changes associated with age, so as to avoid starting untimely treatments that will be difficult to stop. When the use of hypnotics seems necessary (severe insomnia), the parameters to be taken into account are:

- **Dosage:** In our study, 28.1% of doctors reported using half the adult dosage for BZDs, and the same dosage in 34.4% of cases. However, 37.5% did not know the recommended dosage. These attitudes appear to be at odds with the recommendations: only less than a third knew and complied with the recommended dosage (half the adult dose).
- **Duration**: Among the prescriptions proposed in our study, prolonged treatment beyond 1 month was prescribed in 18.75% of cases. On the other hand, it is recommended that hypnotics should only be prescribed for short periods in strict accordance with the authorised indications: from a few days to a maximum of 4 weeks, except for triazolam (2 weeks maximum) including the period of dose reduction.
- **The use of several drugs with a sedative effect** was reported in 6.37% of prescriptions (n=2), and should be avoided.

- **Therapeutic class :**

1. Antihistamines :

These drugs are widely used in the current practice of the participating doctors. (nearly 60%): promethazine (PHENERGAN®) and hydroxyzine (ATARAX®).

However, there is little data on the efficacy of these molecules in insomnia [11], which appears to be rather limited [30]. What's more, the long half-life of some of these molecules facilitates their accumulation in ADSs and in the brain. development of side effects. On the other hand, in addition to their antihistamine effect, several of them have anticholinergic and adrenolytic effects associated with multiple side-effects (dry mucous membranes, constipation, urinary retention, orthostatic hypotension, agitation, blurred vision, cognitive disorders that can lead to confusion in the case of overdoses or in people at risk) [30].

Tolerance effects have also been described, with a rebound effect of insomnia when treatment is stopped [32]. Tls are strongly discouraged in the elderly (according to the Vidal, they should be used with caution in the elderly), and some authors even prohibit them [6].

2. Sedative neuroleptics

In Tunisia, chlorpromazine (largactil®) and levomepromazine (Nozinan®) are available. Their use was noted by 18.75% of prescribers in our study. However, this class has not yet been sufficiently studied in the "insomnia of non-psychotic origin" indication. "In addition, their potentially dangerous side-effects pose problems. What's more, their potentially dangerous side-effects pose problems: fall in blood pressure due to sympathicolysis, anticholinergic effects and extrapyramidal motor effects (tardive dyskinesias) [33].

3. Herbal therapies

Another class widely used by the prescribers in our study (half of them), probably because of the harmless nature often attributed to these molecules. However, there are very few assessments of their efficacy and side-effects. Lime blossom, lemon balm, orange blossom, verbena and hawthorn have no proven efficacy, but they do have some side effects. There is no data to contradict their reputation for safety. The same is true of hawthorn, hops and passionflower, whose safety has been established [34]. Valerian seems to be the only molecule potentially effective on the perceived quality of sleep, although improvement in quantitative sleep measurements has not been demonstrated [35]. In Tunisia, Phytocalm® is available, which acts thanks to a synergy between the three sedative plants lemon balm, valerian and passionflower.

4. Homeopathy:

It is also a class widely used by our participants. SEDATTF PC® is a molecule available on the Tunisian market.

5. Tricyclic antidepressants (TCAs)

Certain antidepressants are often used in low doses to promote sleep. Amitriptyline (ELAVTL®; AMYTRTL®.) is used as a hypnotic, generally in low doses (10 to 50 mg). This prescription was noted in 9.37% of prescribers in our study.Indeed, there is evidence that some tricyclic antidepressants (TCAs) can reduce sleep latency and improve sleep continuity [30]. However, they are generally not the hypnotics of first choice. In fact, TCAs have a high potential for toxicity in the event of overdose and fairly high anticholinergic, antihistaminic and adrenolytic side-effects [30], as well as confusing effects [6]. These treatments do not have an official indication for insomnia [27], and it is imperative that they are contraindicated in ADT.

6. Melatonin

In our study, none of the doctors reported prescribing melatonin. Yet melatonin has its place in the treatment of AS insomnia. Extended-release melatonin, known as Circadin®, obtained its European marketing authorisation in 2008: as monotherapy, two hours before bedtime, in the short-term treatment of primary insomnia in adults aged 55 and over [36]. It has been shown to reduce sleep onset latency, improve sleep quality and morning alertness, and lower core body temperature [37]. Studies have demonstrated the absence of toxicity and severe adverse effects, the absence of cognitive decline, the absence of dependence, even at high doses, and the absence of rebound insomnia or withdrawal symptoms when the drug is discontinued [38].

7. BZDs

In our study, more than half of the participants were used to prescribing BZDs to treat insomnia in AS. This class of drugs has been the most prescribed hypnotics for many years. BZDs reduce sleep latency, the number and duration of nocturnal awakenings, and increase total sleep time and sleep efficiency. They tend to induce light sleep, increasing stages 2 and decreasing stages 3 and 4 [30].

The following table (Table VT) lists the different molecules available, together with some of their pharmacokinetic properties.

Table VI: BZDs: available molecules and pharmacokinetic properties

Class	DCI	Trade name	Elimination half-life		Active metabolites
Class of anxiolytics	Clotiazepam	VERATRAN®	4h	Short	no
	Oxazepam	SERSTA®	8h		no
	lorazepam	TEMESTA®	12h	Tntermé-diaire	no
	alprazolam	XANAX®	12 to 3pm		yes
	bromazepam	LEXOMTL®	20h		yes
	Clobazam	URBANYL®	20 to 50 hours	long	yes
	Diazepam	VALTUM®	32 to 50 hours		yes
	Dipotassium clorazepate	TRANXENE®	40h		yes
	Nordazepam	NORDAZ®	65h		yes
	prazepam	LYSANXTA®	65h		yes
	loflazepate	VTCTAN®	77h		yes
Class of hypnotics	Temazepam	NORMTSON®	5 to 8 h	short	no
	Loprazolam	HAVLANE®	8h		no
	Lormetazepam	NOCTAMTDE®	10h		no
	Estazolam	NUCTALON®	17h		no
	Flunitrazepam	ROHYPNOL®	16 to 35 hours	long	yes
	Nitrazepam	MOGADON®	16 to 48 hours		no
Receptor agonists BZD	Zopiclone	TMOVANE®	5 h	short	no
	Zolpidem	STTLNOX®	2 to 3 hours		no

In fact, the prescription of BZDs in AS must obey certain principles, due to the fragility of the condition:

❖ The half-life of the molecule

In our study, zolpidem (Stilnox®) was the most commonly used drug (21.9%). A previous study looking at the prescription of BZDs in ADS also reported that zolpidem and zopiclone were the most commonly used [3]. Their short elimination half-life (2 to 3 hours) and elimination in the form of inactive metabolites mean that they are both appropriate treatments for ADS. As a general rule, when treatment with BZDs is indicated, the AFSSAPS (Agence Française De Sécurité Sanitaire Des Produits De Santé) recommends giving preference to substances with an intermediate action and no active metabolites (known as short half-lives), as there is a risk of accumulation of the drug or its metabolites (appendix 2). However, we noted significant gaps in doctors' knowledge of this parameter. Indeed, less than half of the prescribers in our study reported using short half-life drugs, and ¼ of them did not know the half-life of the drugs they were using. Furthermore, BZDs with a long half-life (generally accepted threshold > 20 hours) were used in more than a third of cases. It should be emphasised that the half-life of BZDs is a very important parameter to take into account when prescribing them in ADS. It is usually prolonged for two main reasons: the volume of distribution (Vd) is increased and clearance (Cl) is reduced. BZDs with a long half-life are considered inappropriate for AS patients, due to an increased iatrogenic risk [39]. In addition to the "classic" side-effects of BZDs, this category is even more at risk of traumatic falls [40], [41] and increases the risk of hip fractures, particularly with long-term high doses [42], [43].

❖ Contraindications:

It is essential to be aware of them to avoid the sometimes serious complications that can arise in such fragile conditions. However, a quarter of doctors in our study did not recognise them. The contraindications are :

o Severe respiratory insufficiency; sleepapnoea Myasthenia o Severe hepatic insufficiency o Hypersensitivity to benzodiazepines

o Precautions if hepatic/renal insufficiency; machine users; drug addicts

❖ **Duration of treatment**

In the present study, the average length of prescription for BZDs was 34 days (with extremes ranging from 15 days to 3 months). In more than a quarter of cases, the prescription exceeded 30 days. This latter behaviour is rather inconsistent with the recommendations. In fact, BZDs should be prescribed on an ad hoc basis, without exceeding 30 days. Moreover, the HAS recommends that, as soon as treatment is introduced, the doctor should explain to the patient the duration of the treatment and how to stop it, given the risks associated with the treatment (falls and their consequences, cognitive impairment, road accidents, and above all the risk of dependence). In this context, the lack of awareness of these risks among GPs (60%) was another shortcoming observed during our study.

❖ **Drug combinations**

Of the prescriptions proposed that included a BZD (n=11), a combination of drugs was noted in 45.45% of cases (n=5). The various treatments associated with BZDs were: insulin; iron; calcium; risperidone (neuroleptic); aspirin; captopril (antihypertensive); non-steroidal anti-inflammatory drugs; a second BZD. Among these treatments, 2 types of combination are not recommended: BZD/neuroleptics and the combination of two BZDs. Combining BZDs with central nervous system depressants can lead to respiratory depression. On Benzodiazepines should not be combined with sedative antidepressants, H1 antihistamines, barbiturates, other anxiolytics or hypnotics, central antihypertensives, opiate derivatives, neuroleptics or alcohol [44]. Similarly, the combination with antifungal agents (ketoconazole, itraconazole) and macrolide antibiotics (azithromycin; erythromycin) is not recommended [38].

❖ **Withdrawal**

In our study, withdrawal was possible after an average of 50 days of treatment (ranging from 15 days to 6 months). This period exceeded 30 days in half the cases. In fact, the HAS recommends proposing a strategy for discontinuing the use of BZDs and related drugs in all patients with ADHD who have been treated daily for more than 30 days. When initiating discontinuation, the patient's expectations and degree of "attachment" to BZDs should be assessed, using the ECAB questionnaire (Benzodiazepine Attachment Cognitive Scale, appendix 3). Assessing the difficulty of stopping BZDs None of the doctors in this study recognised the ability of ADT to stop taking a BZD. However, this is an essential step before considering weaning, in order to prevent withdrawal syndrome. In fact, when it comes to stopping a BZD, it is important to look for important prognostic factors in order to optimise the approach and adapt it to each patient:

- Duration and dosage of current treatment

Patients who have been taking high doses for a long time are more likely to experience a more severe withdrawal syndrome, to fail to stop taking the drug and to start taking it again.

- Products consumed

Taking several psychotropic drugs at the same time makes it more difficult to stop taking BZDs. The use of a BZD for anxiolytic purposes or the consumption of alcohol before stopping increases the risk of resuming use of BZDs.

- Clinical factors

Severe insomnia and psychological distress are risk factors for the resumption of BZD use. The elderly person's perception of their state of health is a protective factor against the resumption of BZD use.

- Strategies for discontinuing BZDs in elderly patients (appendix 4)

Discontinuation should always be gradual, over a period of several weeks to several months. The rate of dosage reduction varies according to the patient's abilities and the risk of withdrawal syndrome, rebound effect, etc. on discontinuation. As for substitution by another sleeping pill, 12.5% of participants in our study reported using this alternative during and/or after withdrawal. However, according to the French National Authority for Health

(HAS), there are no grounds for proposing drug replacement therapy when stopping BZDs. The emphasis should be on non-medicinal support measures, as long as necessary.

In our study, BZDs were stopped in an average of 47 days, with extremes ranging from 7 days to 6 months. In 18.75% of cases, withdrawal took place in less than 30 days, and was therefore relatively rapid. However, the HAS insists that cessation should always be gradual, and can usually be achieved in 4 to 10 weeks on an outpatient basis (e.g. an initial reduction in dosage of around 25% in the first week). However, long-term users or those receiving high doses of BZDs or related drugs may need to stop taking them over several months.

Some authors suggest replacing short half-life benzodiazepines with longer half-life benzodiazepines to reduce withdrawal symptoms [45]. Other drugs have been shown to be useful during withdrawal, such as carbamazepine, sodium valproate and gabapentin, However, a meta-analysis shows that tapering with medication is no more effective than tapering alone, and that tapering is more effective than rapid tapering with medication [46].

- Withdrawal syndrome (WS)

Diagnosis of SS

All chronic users of BZDs are at risk of withdrawal syndrome if they stop taking them suddenly, whether accidentally or not.

In elderly patients, when cessation is not planned and monitored, withdrawal syndrome is under-diagnosed, because the symptoms are attributed to age or other associated illnesses. In fact, in our study, we noted marked gaps in doctors' knowledge of both the diagnosis and management of this syndrome.

In fact, more than half the doctors did not recognise the symptoms of withdrawal syndrome. The two signs reported were increased insomnia and agitation. These were signs of moderate intensity. In addition, other more serious symptoms may also be seen (haemodynamic and neuro-vegetative disturbances) (appendix 5).

management of the SS : Here too, the participants' knowledge was lacking.

More than half had not suggested any course of action.Among the solutions, a return to the previous dose was proposed in 3.12% of cases. This is the recommendation of the HAS in the presence of non-serious signs during the tapering phase of BZDs or related drugs. The drug should then be withdrawn more gradually. However, once the BZDs have been completely stopped, it is recommended that treatment should never be resumed. In most cases, information and psychological support should be provided until the signs have disappeared.In addition, 3.12% of doctors reported the need to look for anxiety and/or depression. In fact, if the signs of SS are more severe or persistent, the HAS recommends a diagnostic re-evaluation for specific treatment in the context of a precise diagnosis (depression, anxiety disorders, proven insomnia, etc.).Some participants had reported prescribing a symptomatic treatment during SS, in this case a beta-blocker. Propanolol has been tested in this context in previous studies, but appears to have a limited impact on the severity of the withdrawal syndrome. Moreover, one study showed that gradual discontinuation alone was more effective than abrupt discontinuation with propanolol [47]. Finally, if the patient shows serious signs of BZD withdrawal syndrome (confusion, hallucinations, impaired alertness, convulsions, coma), he or she should be admitted to hospital for symptomatic treatment.

5. CONCLUSION

Insomnia, defined as difficulties in falling asleep or staying asleep, or non-restorative sleep, is the most common sleep disorder in the elderly. The management of insomnia must take account of the physiological changes associated with age, the greater frequency of co-morbidities and multi-medication. Hypnotics must therefore be prescribed with caution, as they are particularly vulnerable to falls in the elderly, which can sometimes lead to serious complications, as well as cognitive impairment and road accidents. As a result, management must comply with international recommendations in order to minimise these risks. The aim of this study was to assess GP practices in the management of insomnia in the elderly and to compare them with international recommendations.For this reason, we conducted an observational, cross-sectional and descriptive study among general practitioners in the Sfax region, over a period of 2 months (January and February 2016). We invited these doctors to take part in our survey by sending them a questionnaire via their emails, which they completed anonymously. Out of a total of 348 e-mails sent, we received only 32 responses, i.e. a rate of 9.2%.Among the participants, 62.5% reported that they are very often or often called upon by elderly patients consulting them for insomnia. Before prescribing a hypnotic, 65.6% of doctors reported that they usually recommend a few healthy dietary habits. However, 71.9% thought that these rules were rarely or never effective. When it came to prescribing sleeping pills, only 34.4% of doctors reported that they found it easy to prescribe a hypnotic for an elderly patient. The classes most commonly used were: BZDs (59.37%), antihistamines (59.37%), homeopathic treatments (56.25%) and phytotherapy (50%). In addition, 40.6% thought that they were in control of prescribing these hypnotics, which they did in accordance with recommendations in ¼ of cases. However, 46.9% said they knew nothing about these recommendations.

The sample prescriptions proposed by the participants showed that 18.75% of them did not comply with international recommendations for the duration of treatment.As for the prescription of BZDs, contrary to HAS recommendations, long half-life compounds were used in 37.48% of cases. Similarly, contrary to these recommendations, 34.4% used the same dosage as adults, and 37.5% did not know the recommended dosage.Knowledge of the diagnosis and management of BZD withdrawal syndrome was also lacking. Among prescribers, 56.25% did not recognise the symptoms of this syndrome, and 59.37% had not reported any behaviour in the event of its occurrence. Our study has shown that the prescription of hypnotic treatment in the elderly follows a logical approach to care, after a precise diagnosis, taking into account psychiatric and somatic comorbidities, precautions for use and contraindications. Our study highlighted a number of shortcomings in the management of insomnia in elderly patients in general practice. There is a need for more training in this area.

BIBLIOGRAPHY

[1] Patel D, Steinberg J, Patel P. Tnsomnia in the Elderly: A Review. J Clin Sleep Med. 2018;14(6):1017-1024.

[2] Office parlementaire d'évaluation des politiques de santé. Report on the proper use of psychotropic drugs. 2006.

[3] Emmanuelle SAGER. Thesis: long-term benzodiazepines in the elderly. Lorraine, October 2013

[4] Lindsey PL. Psychotropic medication use among older adults: what all nurses need to know. J Gerontol Nurs. 2009;35(9):28-38. doi:10.3928/00989134-20090731-01

[5] Haute Autorité de Santé: Améliorer la prescription des psychotropes chez la personne âgée. Anxiety. 2008 progress report

[6] T. Montemayor. Sleep in the elderly: evolution, disorders and management. Médecine du sommeil 2008; 5(15), March 2008:5-9

[7] Zeitzer JM, Daniels JE, Duffy JF, et al. Do plasma melatonin concentrations decline with age? Am J Med 1999 ; 107: 432-436.

[8] Rodenbeck A, Hajak G. Neuroendocrine dysregulation in primary insomnia. Rev Neurol 2001; 157(11Pt2): 57-61

[9] Bliwise DL. Normal Aging. Tn: Kryger MH, Roth T, Dement WC, eds. Principles and practice of sleep medicine 3rd edition. Philadelphia: Saunders.2000: 26-42

[1O] Duffy JF, Dijk DJ, Klerman EB, et al. Later endogenous circadian temperature rhythms to an earlier wake time in older people.Am J Physiol 1998; 275: R1478-R1487

[11] Tiberge M. Sleep in extreme situations. Hegel 2019;3:240.
[12] Vecchierini-Blineau MF. Modification of sleep with age. La Revue de Gériatrie 2002; 27: 5-12.
[13] Goldenberg F.Sleep in normal aging.Neurophysiol Clin 1991; 21: 267-279
[14] Vecchierini-Blineau MF. Le sommeil du sujet âgé. Bulletin veille et sommeil 1992 ;1:10-14
[15] Dijk DJ, Duffy JF, Riel E et al. Ageing and the circadian and homeostatic regulation of human sleep during forced desynchrony of rest, melatonin and temperature rhythms. J Physiology 1999;516: 611-7
[16] Ficca G,Gori S, Ktonas P, et al. The organization of rapid eye movement is impaired in the elderly. Neurosci Lett 1999; 275: 219-221

[17] Billiard M, Dauvilliers Y. Tnsomnia. EMC-Neurologie. 2004:209-222
[18] Perilliat T, Sebbane D, Sebbane G. Gériatrie et gérontopsychiatrie - Les aides mémoire du diplôme d'Etat d'infirmier. TFST Mémo 17, 2003

[19] Mizrahi A, Mizrahi A. Consumers of sleeping pills. Gérontologie et société 2006; 29(116):207-214

[20] Hervy MP, Molitor MB, Beguin V, Chahbenderian L, Farah S. Gérontologie gérontopsychiatrie 2019. Elsevier / Masson

[21] Report on the theme of sleep. Ministry of Health and Solidarity - Dec. 2006
[22] Haute Autorité de Santé. Améliorer la Prescription des psychotropes Chez le sujet âgé, Propositions d'actions concertées, October 2007.

[23] Haute Autorité de Santé. Modalités d'arrêt des benzodiazépines et médicaments apparentés chez le patient âgé, Professional recommendations. October 2007

[24] Haute Autorité de Santé. Prise en charge de l'insomnie en médecine générale. Professional recommendations. 2007

[25] High Authority for Health. Stopping the use of benzodiazepines and related drugs: an approach for outpatient GPs, June 2015

[26] Haute Autorité de Santé. What place for benzodiazepines in insomnia? February 2015

[27] Haute Autorité de Santé. Prise en charge du patient adulte se plaignant d'insomnie en médecine générale. December 2006

[28] Perivier S, Mendes A, Heyrani Nobari B, Ammane H, Cervena K, Perrig S, Zekry D. Practical approach to insomnia in geriatrics: from complaint to treatment. Rev Med Suisse 2015; 11: 2098-103

[29] Trwin MR, Cole JC, Nicassio PM. Comparative meta-analysis of behavioral interventions for insomnia and their efficacy in middle-aged adults and in older adults 55+ years of age. Health Psychol. 2006;25(1):3-14. doi:10.1037/0278-6133.25.1.3

[30] Goulet J, Chaloult L, Ngô TL. Practice guide for the assessment andcognitive-behavioural treatment of insomnia.Jean -tcc montreal 2018.

[31] Harsora P, Kessmann J. Nonpharmacologic management of chronic insomnia. Am Fam Physician. 2009;79(2):125-130.

[32] Morin CM, Benca R. Chronic insomnia [published correction appears in Lancet. 2012 Apr 21;379(9825):1488]. Lancet. 2012;379(9821):1129-1141. doi:10.1016/S0140-6736(11)60750-2

[33] Hatzingera M, Hattenschwilerb J. Treatment of sleep disorders. Forum Med Suisse 2001;11:271-276

[34] Insomnia complaints: A place for traditional herbal medicine. La revue Prescrire2005; 25(258): 110

[35] Fernandez-San-Martin MT, Masa-Font R, Palacios-Soler L, Sancho-G6mez P, Calb6- Caldentey C, Flores-Mateo G. Effectiveness of Valerian on insomnia: a meta-analysis of randomized placebo-controlled trials. Sleep Med. 2010;11(6):505-511. doi:10.1016/ j.sleep.2009.12.009

[36] Srinivasan V, Pandi-Perumal SR, Trahkt T, et al. Melatonin and melatonergic drugs on sleep: possible mechanisms of action. Tnt J Neurosci. 2009;119(6):821-846. doi:10.1080/00207450802328607

[37] Vecchierini MF, Kilic-Huck U, Quera-Salva MA, members of the SFRMS consensus group. Melatonin (MEL) and its use in neurological pathologies and insomnia: recommendations of the French Society of Sleep Research and Medicine (SFRMS). Médecine du Sommeil. 2021;18(2): 70-89.

[38] Tuft C, Matar E, Menczel Schrire Z, Grunstein RR, Yee BJ, Hoyos CM. Current Tnsights into the Risks of Using Melatonin as a Treatment for Sleep Disorders in Older Adults. Clin Tnterv Aging. 2023;18:49-59.

[39] Caisse Nationale de l'Assurance Maladie des Travailleurs Salariés. Choix d'une benzodiazépine chez le sujet âgé de plus de 65 ans et polypathologique ou après 75 ans. Paris: CNAMTS; 2008.

[40] Beauchet O, Annweiler C, Hureaux-Huynh R. Medications and falls in the elderly. Ann Gérontol 2008;1:47-52

[41] Berdot S, Bertrand M, Dartigues JF, et al. Tnappropriate medication use and risk of falls--a prospective study in a large community-dwelling elderly cohort. BMC Geriatr. 2009;9:30. Published 2009 Jul 23. doi:10.1186/1471-2318-9-30

[42] Wagner AK, Zhang F, Soumerai SB, et al. Benzodiazepine use and hip fractures in the elderly: who is at greatest risk? Arch Tntern Med 2004 ;164 (14):1567-72

[43] Schneeweiss S, Wang PS. Claims data studies of sedative-hypnotics and hip fractures in older people: exploring residual confounding using survey information. J Am Geriatr Soc 2005;53(6):948-54

[44] Perlemuter L. Perlemuter G. Guide de thérapeutique. Masson, 7th edition, 2013; 1577

[45] O'connor KP, Marchand A, Brousseau L, et al. Evaluation of a benzodiazepine withdrawal program. Santé Mentale au Québec. 2003; 28(2): 121-148

[46] Parr JM, Kavanagh DJ, Cahill L, et al. Effectiveness of current treatment approaches for benzodiazepine discontinuation: a meta-analysis. Addiction. 2009; 104(1): 13-24

[47] Schweizer E, Rickels K. Benzodiazepine dependence and withdrawal: a review of the syndrome and its clinical management. Acta Psychiatr Scand Suppl. 1998; 393: 95-101

APPENDIXES

APPENDIX 1 :

treatment of insomnia in the elderly

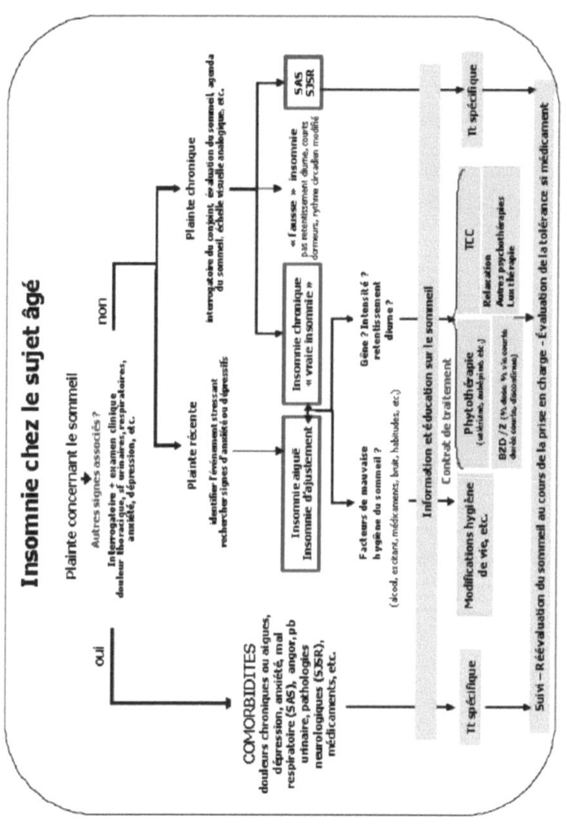

APPENDIX 2

BENZO Juin 2008

Choix d'une benzodiazépine[1] chez le sujet âgé de plus de 65 ans et polypathologique ou après 75 ans

Lorsqu'un traitement par benzodiazépine est indiqué, *l'Agence Française de Sécurité Sanitaire des Produits de Santé recommande de privilégier les substances d'action intermédiaire et sans métabolite actif (dites à "demi-vie courte"), car* ***il existe un risque d'accumulation du médicament ou de ses métabolites lors de prises répétées.***

→ À privilégier : benzodiazépines à "demi-vie courte" (< 20 heures)[2]

Nom commercial	Molécule	Demi-vie[3] (heure)	Métabolite actif cliniquement pertinent
Classe des hypnotiques			
STILNOX®	**Zolpidem**	2h30	non
IMOVANE®	**Zopiclone**	5	non
NORMISON®	**Témazépam**	5 à 8	non
HAVLANE®	**Loprazolam**	8	non
NOCTAMIDE®	**Lormétazépam**	10	non
NUCTALON®	**Estazolam**	17	non
Classe des anxiolytiques			
VERATRAN®	**Clotiazépam**	4	non
SERESTA®	**Oxazépam**	8	non
TEMESTA®	**Lorazépam**	10 à 20	non
XANAX®	**Alprazolam**	10 à 20	non

⚠ À éviter : benzodiazépines à "demi-vie longue" (≥ 20 heures)[2]

Nom commercial	Molécule	Demi-vie[3] (heure)	Métabolite actif cliniquement pertinent
Classe des hypnotiques			
ROHYPNOL®	**Flunitrazépam**	16 à 35	oui
MOGADON®	**Nitrazépam**	16 à 48	non
Classe des anxiolytiques			
LEXOMIL®	**Bromazépam**	20	non
URBANYL®	**Clobazam**	20	oui
VALIUM®	**Diazépam**	32 à 47	oui
VICTAN®	**Ethyle loflazépate**	77	non
LYSANXIA®	**Prazépam**	30 à 150	oui
NORDAZ®	**Nordazépam**	30 à 150	oui
TRANXENE® NOCTRAN®[4]	**Clorazépate dipotassique**	30 à 150	oui

[1] Liste non exhaustive, concernant les benzodiazépines et apparentés (agonistes des récepteurs aux benzodiazépines)

[2] Définition adoptée dans une étude conduite dans la cohorte des 3 cités (Nathalie Lechevallier-Michel et al : *European Journal of Clinical Pharmacology 2004*)

[3] Demi-vie mesurée chez l'adulte

[4] Association de Clorazépate dipotassique et de deux neuroleptiques

Fiche réalisée avec la contribution du Pr J. Doucet et du Pr S. Legrain, établie en accord avec la HAS.

Juin 2008 - SG/DGM/Diag1

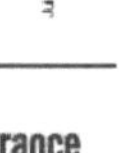

l'Assurance Maladie

APPENDIX 3: ECAB scale

Échelle cognitive d'attachement aux benzodiazépines
(attribuer 1 point en cas de réponse « vrai »,
sauf question 10 = 1 point en cas de réponse « faux »)

Les questions ci-dessous concernent certaines idées que vous pouvez avoir sur les médicaments **tranquillisants** et/ou **somnifères** que vous prenez.

Si une proposition correspond à ce que vous pensez, cochez la case « vrai » ; cochez la case « faux » dans le cas contraire.

Il est indispensable de répondre à **toutes** les propositions avec **une seule** réponse « vrai » ou « faux », même si vous n'êtes pas très sûr(e) de votre réponse.

Nom du médicament concerné : ....

		Vrai	Faux
1.	Où que j'aille, j'ai besoin d'avoir ce médicament avec moi................	☐1	☐0
2.	Ce médicament est pour moi comme une drogue	☐1	☐0
3.	Je pense souvent que je ne pourrai jamais arrêter ce médicament...	☐1	☐0
4.	J'évite de dire à mes proches que je prends ce médicament...........	☐1	☐0
5.	J'ai l'impression de prendre beaucoup trop de ce médicament.........	☐1	☐0
6.	J'ai parfois peur à l'idée de manquer de ce médicament..................	☐1	☐0
7.	Lorsque j'arrête ce médicament, je me sens très malade.................	☐1	☐0
8.	Je prends ce médicament parce que je ne peux plus m'en passer.	☐1	☐0
9.	Je prends ce médicament parce que je vais mal quand j'arrête........	☐1	☐0
10.	Je ne prends ce médicament que lorsque j'en ressens le besoin......	☐0	☐1

Le questionnaire ECAB est constitué de 10 items cotés 1 ou 0. Le score total a questionnaire est obtenu par la somme des points aux différents items. Un score ≥ 6 perme de différencier les patients dépendants des patients non dépendants avec une sensibilit de 94 % et une spécificité de 81 %.

HAS / Service des recommandations professionnelles / Octobre 2007

APPENDIX 4 :

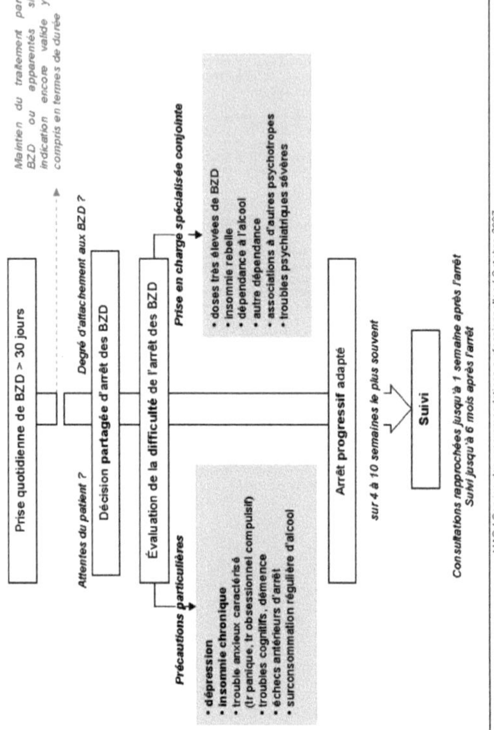

ARRÊT DES BENZODIAZÉPINES ET APPARENTÉS CHEZ LE PATIENT DE PLUS DE 65 ANS
DÉMARCHE DU MÉDECIN TRAITANT EN AMBULATOIRE
Prise quotidienne de BZD > 30 jours
Maintien du traitement par BZD ou apparentés si indication encore valide y compris en termes de durée
Attentes du patient ?
Degré d'attachement aux BZD ?
Décision partagée d'arrêt des BZD
Évaluation de la difficulté de l'arrêt des BZD
Précautions particulières
• dépression
• insomnie chronique
• trouble anxieux caractérisé
(tr panique, tr obsessionnel compulsif)
• troubles cognitifs, démence
• échecs antérieurs d'arrêt
• surconsommation régulière d'alcool
Prise en charge spécialisée conjointe
• doses très élevées de BZD
• insomnie rebelle
• dépendance à l'alcool
• autre dépendance
• associations à d'autres psychotropes
• troubles psychiatriques sévères
Arrêt progressif adapté
sur 4 à 10 semaines le plus souvent
Suivi
Consultations rapprochées jusqu'à 1 semaine après l'arrêt
Suivi jusqu'à 6 mois après l'arrêt
HAS / Service des recommandations professionnelles / Octobre 2007

APPENDIX 5:

benzodiazepine withdrawal symptoms

Intensité	Signes
Modérée	Agitation
	Anxiété, nervosité
	Céphalées
	Diaphorèse
	Diarrhée
	Dysphorie
	Étourdissement
	Faiblesses ou raideurs musculaires
	Fatigue
	Goût métallique dans la bouche
	Impatience
	Insomnie
	Irritabilité
	Léthargie
	Manque de motivation
	Perte d'appétit
	Sensibilité accrue aux bruits et aux odeurs
	Trouble de concentration
Sévère	Cauchemars
	Confusion
	Convulsions (rare)
	Délire
	Dépersonnalisation
	Distorsion perceptuelle
	Fasciculations
	Hypotension orthostatique
	Mauvaise coordination ou incoordination motrice
	Nausées, vomissements
	Tachycardie, palpitations
	Tremblements
	Vertiges

[7] Signes le plus souvent rapportés lors de l'arrêt graduel des BZD chez des patients qui prenan de 1 an.

CONTENTS

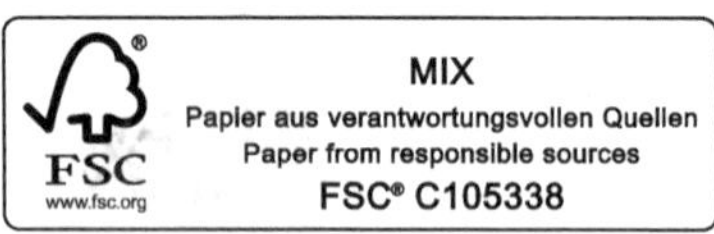

Printed by Books on Demand GmbH, Norderstedt / Germany